Paxlovid

The Revolutionary Antiviral for COVID-19 and Beyond

Dr Ronald L. Bell

TABLE OF CONTENTS

PAXLOVID

Paxlovid is a medicine used to treat mild to moderate COVID-19 instances brought on by the SARS-CoV-2 virus. It is an oral antiviral medication created by Pfizer in association with the pharmaceuticals maker AstraZeneca. In December 2021, the U.S. Food and Drug Administration (FDA) granted Paxlovid an Emergency Use Authorization (EUA), and other governments had granted similar authorizations.

These are Paxlovid's salient characteristics:

Active Components:

Nirmatrelvir and ritonavir are the two active components that make up

Paxlovid. Together, these two medications prevent the SARS-CoV-2 virus from replicating.

2. Action Mechanism:

The primary protease (Mpro) of the SARS-CoV-2 virus is the target of the protease inhibitor nirmatrelvir. The replication of the virus requires this protease.

By blocking the CYP3A4 enzyme, which metabolizes nirmatrelvir, ritonavir is used in conjunction with nirmatrelvir to increase the bioavailability and effectiveness of nirmatrelvir in the body.

3. Significance

Paxlovid is approved for the treatment of mild to moderate COVID-19 in patients 12 years of age and older who weigh at least 40 kilograms (88 pounds), according to the FDA.

It is specifically advised for those who tested positive for SARS-CoV-2 and are at a high risk of the disease progressing to a severe stage. Those at risk for a severe COVID-19 include the elderly, people with underlying medical issues, and others.

4. Administration and Dosage:

Paxlovid pills are taken orally to provide the medication.

Three pills of nirmatrelvir/ritonavir, each containing 150 mg/100 mg, are typically taken twice daily for a total of five days when using Paxlovid. Nirmatrelvir and ritonavir are combined at a daily dose of 600 mg and 400 mg, respectively.

5. Result:

evaluating the drug's safety profile, dose, and mode of metabolism.

Participants: A small number of healthy volunteers or those with the condition the medicine is intended to treat are usually included in these trials.

Paxlovid: During this stage, researchers would have assessed the tolerability of nirmatrelvir/ritonavir and determined whether there were any immediate safety issues.

2. Clinical Trials in Phase 2:

Goal: Phase 2 trials build on the safety information gained in Phase 1 and start to evaluate the drug's efficacy.

Participants: Phase 2 trials feature a larger number of individuals with the targeted ailment.

Paxlovid: During this stage, scientists would have begun to investigate whether Paxlovid had any therapeutic impact on COVID-19, particularly in terms of symptom relief and viral load reduction.

3. Clinical Trials in Phase 3:

The purpose of phase 3 trials is to further evaluate the safety and effectiveness of the medication through larger, more thorough research. Thousands of people frequently participate in them.

Participants: To better understand how the medicine functions in various demographics, phase 3 trials include a variety of patients.

Paxlovid: In these studies, researchers looked at outcomes like hospitalization rates, symptom alleviation, and general outcomes to determine the drug's effect on COVID-19 in practical situations.

4. RCTs: Randomized Controlled Trials

Design: Randomized controlled trials (RCTs), the industry standard for clinical research, make up a large portion of Phase 3 trials. In RCTs, patients are randomized at random to receive either the medication (Paxlovid) or a placebo, guaranteeing that the findings are not skewed.

RCTs are frequently double-blind, which means neither the patients nor the researchers are aware of whether they are receiving the real medication or a placebo. By doing this, reporting and assessment bias is reduced.

Regulatory Acceptance:

Outcome: Paxlovid was assessed by regulatory organizations including the U.S. Food and Drug Administration

(FDA) and other international counterparts based on the findings from these clinical trials.

Paxlovid was granted an Emergency Use Authorization (EUA) by the FDA in December 2021, which meant it was proven to be safe and effective enough to be utilized during the COVID-19 pandemic.

Real-World Information:

Post-Marketing Surveillance: Following approval, medications like Paxlovid continue to be checked for efficacy and safety in actual clinical settings.

It's vital to remember that clinical trial data is frequently published in medical journals, and these publications would contain detailed outcomes. Additionally, Paxlovid clinical trial procedures are subject to strict ethical and regulatory scrutiny to safeguard research participants' rights and safety. The outcomes of these trials give medical practitioners the knowledge they need to choose wisely whether to utilize Paxlovid to treat COVID-19.

DISTRIBUTION AND AVAILABILITY OF PAXLOVID

Paxlovid, a drug used to treat COVID-19, must be distributed and made readily available if it is to be utilized effectively in the fight against the pandemic. I'll give a thorough description of Paxlovid's distribution and accessibility as of my most recent knowledge update in September 2021. It's crucial to remember that this material may have changed since then, therefore for the most recent details, please refer to current sources and recommendations.

Emergency Use Authorization (EUA) and Regulatory Approvals:

Regulatory Authorities: In order for Paxlovid to be distributed and made accessible, it must first gain regulatory approval from health authorities in various nations. For instance, the U.S. Food and Drug Administration (FDA) granted Paxlovid an Emergency Use Authorization (EUA) in December 2021. Other health agencies in many nations have issued similar authorizations or licenses.

2. Production and Manufacturing:

Pharmaceutical Firms: Paxlovid is produced by pharmaceutical firms that have the necessary licenses. Strict quality control procedures are used during the manufacturing process to guarantee the medication's effectiveness and safety.

Production Scaling Up: In response to the COVID-19 epidemic, Paxlovid production is being increased to keep up with demand on a global scale. This includes developing supply chains and increasing production capacity.

Networks of Distribution

Paxlovid is distributed both domestically and internationally through a network of healthcare supply chains. These networks make sure the medication gets to pharmacies, medical facilities, and other authorized distribution places.

Allocation Strategies: Some nations have put in place allocation strategies to provide Paxlovid priority distribution to regions with higher COVID-19 prevalence or to high-risk groups such the elderly and people with underlying medical issues.

4. Accessibility in Medical Facilities:

Hospitals and Clinics: Paxlovid is frequently provided in healthcare settings including hospitals and clinics where COVID-19 patients receive medical attention. For those who have a high chance of having severe COVID-19, this is extremely crucial.

Paxlovid may eventually be made available in outpatient settings, enabling people with mild to moderate COVID-19 to receive therapy.

5. Equity and Access:

Global Access: It is difficult to guarantee Paxlovid's availability everywhere. To provide the medication to nations with scarce resources, international cooperation and support are crucial.

Equity Issues: It is a problem to make sure that everyone has access to Paxlovid, especially for underprivileged groups and nations with limited resources. There are initiatives to reduce these discrepancies.

Monitoring and reporting, or 6.

Pharmacovigilance: Following distribution, Paxlovid is continually checked for efficacy and safety by pharmacovigilance programs. This entails keeping track of and disclosing any negative outcomes or medication-related side effects.

7. Changing Accessibility:

Supply Chain concerns: Just like with other COVID-19 therapies and vaccinations, Paxlovid's accessibility may be impacted by supply chain concerns such a lack of raw materials and shipping problems.

Regulatory updates: As new information becomes available, availability may vary. Regulatory authorities also revise their guidelines in light of the developing knowledge of COVID-19 and its management.

Healthcare professionals and the general public should be kept up to date on Paxlovid's distribution and accessibility via authorized channels and healthcare authorities. Availability may differ by location, and access may be constrained by particular standards and requirements set by regional health authorities.

IMPACT OF PAXLOVID ON HOSPITALIZATION AND MORTALITY

Nirmatrelvir and ritonavir, which make up Paxlovid, have proven to be extremely beneficial in lowering hospitalization and mortality in patients with mild to moderate COVID-19. Here is a thorough description of how Paxlovid affects these important results:

Clinical studies and actual data

Clinical trial results and real-world research are the main sources of information used to determine how successful Paxlovid is at lowering hospitalization and mortality.
Early Treatment Is Important:

Early on in the COVID-19 course is when paxlovid is most effective. It functions by preventing the SARS-CoV-2 virus from replicating, lowering viral load, and potentially lessening the severity of the illness.

3. Decreased Hospitalization Risk:

Paxlovid dramatically lowers the likelihood of hospitalization in those with mild to moderate COVID-19, according to clinical research.

For instance, Paxlovid revealed an 88% decrease in the incidence of COVID-19-related hospitalization or mortality compared to placebo in the EPIC-HR (Evaluation of Protease Inhibition for COVID-19 in High-incidence Patients) trial.

4. Decreased Mortality Risk:

Additionally, paxlovid has been linked to a decline in mortality in COVID-19 patients.

Paxlovid showed an 89% decrease in the risk of death from any cause when compared to placebo in the same EPIC-HR trial.

5. Protection for Populations at High Risk:

For high-risk groups that are more susceptible to severe COVID-19, like the elderly and people with underlying medical issues, paxlovid is especially beneficial.

One of the main objectives of COVID-19 therapy is to prevent hospitalization and mortality in these populations.

6. Decreased viral load

In conclusion, Paxlovid, especially when given early in the course of the disease, has shown significant effectiveness in lowering the risk of hospitalization and death in people with mild to moderate COVID-19. Healthcare practitioners should follow the most recent advice and recommendations from regulatory bodies and health authorities as its accessibility and usage may differ by region.

SIDE EFFECTS AND SAFETY PROFILE FOR PAXLOVID

Like any drug, paxlovid has a distinct set of possible side effects as well as a safety profile that patients and healthcare professionals should be aware of. The adverse effects and safety concerns of Paxlovid are explained in detail below:

1. Typical Adverse Effects:

Gastrointestinal Symptoms: Nausea and diarrhea are two of the most frequent Paxlovid side effects.
Rash on the skin has also been described as a negative effect.
2. Safety Overview:

Clinical Trials: Clinical trials involving thousands of individuals have assessed the safety of Paxlovid. These tests evaluated its general safety, medication interactions, and side effects.

Paxlovid was given an emergency use authorization (EUA) by the U.S. Food and Drug Administration (FDA), as well as equivalent authorizations in other nations, based on a positive evaluation of its safety and effectiveness.

Drug Reactions: 3.

Ritonavir, a component of Paxlovid, is used to increase the bioavailability of nirmatrelvir, the primary active ingredient. Healthcare professionals should evaluate a patient's current medication list to look for any drug interactions because ritonavir can interact with other drugs.

4. Reactions to Allergies:

Paxlovid allergic responses can happen, albeit being uncommon. If patients have symptoms like hives, itching, swelling of the face or throat, or trouble breathing, they should consult a doctor right away.

5. Liver (Hepatic) Safety:

Liver function may be impacted by some protease inhibitors, including ritonavir in Paxlovid. Patients need to be kept an eye out for symptoms of liver issues including jaundice (a yellowing of the skin or eyes), dark urine, or lingering abdominal pain.

6. Nursing and pregnancy:

Paxlovid's safety for use during pregnancy and breast-feeding is not entirely known. When thinking about prescribing it to women who are pregnant or nursing, healthcare professionals should assess the potential advantages and disadvantages.

7. Safety Measures for Particular Populations:

Pediatric Patients: It is unknown whether Paxlovid is safe and effective for use in children who are under a certain age and weight.

Patients who are elderly: Because elderly patients may be more vulnerable to some side effects, careful monitoring is advised.

Patients with considerable Liver Impairment: Patients who have considerable liver impairment may need dose changes or extra supervision.

8. Disclosure of Side Effects:

It is advised that healthcare professionals and patients notify the appropriate regulatory authorities of any Paxlovid side effects or adverse events. This aids in continuing medication safety monitoring.

9. Ongoing Inspection:

Following regulatory approval, pharmacovigilance programs continue to check the safety of drugs like Paxlovid in actual clinical settings.

10. Risks vs. Benefits:

The potential advantages of Paxlovid in lessening the severity of COVID-19 and averting hospitalization and death must be weighed against the dangers, which include side effects and medication interactions.

Those who are considering Paxlovid as a COVID-19 treatment should have frank and knowledgeable discussions with their medical professionals. To make sure Paxlovid is a safe and suitable alternative for them, patients should be open and honest about their medical history, current drugs, and any allergies. In addition, patients should use Paxlovid according to the advice of their doctor and watch out for any odd symptoms or adverse effects when taking the drug.

PAXLOVID IN POPULATIONS AT HIGH RISK

Paxlovid, a drug used to treat COVID-19, is crucial in the control of the illness in high-risk populations. People in high-risk populations are those who are more likely to suffer serious consequences if they get COVID-19. The elderly, people with preexisting medical illnesses, and people who have particular risk factors are frequently included in these demographics. Here is a thorough justification of Paxlovid's application and significance in high-risk populations:

Prime Populations at Risk:

People in high-risk populations are those who are more likely to catch COVID-19 and experience a severe illness, require hospitalization, or pass away. Age, underlying medical disorders, immunosuppression, and other vulnerabilities all contribute to this elevated risk.

2. The Value of Early Intervention:

When given early in COVID-19, ideally within the first few days of symptom manifestation, pax ovid is most helpful.

When experiencing COVID-19 symptoms, high-risk persons should contact their doctor right once and go through testing to determine their diagnosis.

3. Lowering Mortality and Hospitalization:

Using Paxlovid in high-risk populations is primarily intended to lower the risk of hospitalization and mortality.

Paxlovid can dramatically reduce the likelihood of severe outcomes in people with mild to moderate COVID-19, particularly when treatment is started early, according to clinical trials and real-world evidence.

4. Concentrating on Coexisting Health Conditions

People in high-risk populations frequently have underlying medical issues such diabetes, heart disease, respiratory problems, and immunosuppressive illnesses.

By directly attacking the SARS-CoV-2 virus, Paxlovid's antiviral effect aids in the regulation of viral replication and may help people with these circumstances avoid developing severe illness.

5. Complement to Vaccination:

The most effective method of avoiding COVID-19, particularly severe instances, is still immunization; however, not all members of high-risk populations will always develop a robust immune response to vaccines.

When combined with immunization, paxlovid can give an extra layer of defense against illnesses that emerge suddenly.

6. Factors to Consider for Older Adults:

Elderly people are most susceptible to negative effects from COVID-19. For older persons, paxlovid may be a beneficial therapy option.

Paxlovid may be taken into account by medical professionals as part of an all-encompassing COVID-19 management strategy for older people.

7. Customized Treatment Programs:

To choose the best course of action, healthcare professionals consider each patient's risk factors, current health, and stage of COVID-19 infection.

Depending on the circumstances, paxlovid may be used either alone or in conjunction with other medicines.

8. Follow-Up and Monitoring:

Paxlovid-treated high-risk patients need to have their conditions constantly watched for any changes.

Regular check-ins and follow-up sessions may be scheduled by healthcare professionals to make sure the treatment is working and to address any new concerns.

9. Access and Equity:

It is crucial to provide high-risk populations, notably underserved communities, fair access to Paxlovid. Reaching out to vulnerable groups and giving them access to this treatment option should be a priority.

10. Ongoing Investigation:

Paxlovid's function in high-risk populations is still being studied, along with the drug's long-term effectiveness and safety.

Paxlovid is an effective technique for lowering COVID-19's severe results, particularly in high-risk patients. However, healthcare professionals that take into account each patient's individual medical history, risk factors, and the developing landscape of COVID-19 treatments and guidelines should direct its use.

COVID-19 AND PAXLOVID VARIANTS

Given how quickly the virus is developing, Paxlovid, a drug used to treat COVID-19, and its effect on SARS-CoV-2 variations must be taken into account. The virus's virulence, capacity for transmission, and susceptibility to treatment responses may all vary. The significance of Paxlovid in relation to COVID-19 variations is explained in more detail below:

1. SARS-CoV-2 variants

The virus that causes COVID-19, SARS-CoV-2, has the capacity to mutate throughout time, resulting in the formation of variations.

The spike protein, which the virus uses to enter human cells, may have genetic modifications in some forms, which could have an impact on the virus's transmissibility and how it interacts with drugs and vaccinations.

2. Effect on Antiviral Therapy:

The effectiveness of antiviral medications like Paxlovid could conceivably be impacted by virus variations that alter the spike protein. Changes to the spike protein may affect how well antiviral medications limit viral replication and so affect how susceptible the virus is to them.

3. Research on variations

The effectiveness of Paxlovid and other antiviral medications against various SARS-CoV-2 mutations is currently being studied.

Laboratory tests can shed light on how well these medications work against particular variations based on their genetic make-up.

4. Possible Modifications:

To continue to be effective against novel variations, antiviral medications like Paxlovid may require modifications or adaptations.

Pharmaceutical businesses and researchers continuously track variant developments to see whether medicine formulations need to be changed.

Impact on Public Health, Number 5

The possible impact of variants on the efficacy of treatments emphasizes the significance of public health initiatives like immunization, which can offer broader protection against several variants.

Combination therapies, or 6.

To improve the efficacy of treatment against various variations, healthcare providers may occasionally consider combination therapies that involve multiple medications with distinct mechanisms of action.

7. Sequencing and surveillance

Understanding how the virus is changing and whether it affects treatment and vaccine responses requires ongoing surveillance and genetic sequencing of SARS-CoV-2 variants.

Monitoring identifies different types of problems and provides information for public health actions.

8. Quick Reaction

One of the most important aspects of pandemic response is the capacity to swiftly alter medications like Paxlovid to address new variations.

Pharmaceutical firms and regulatory organizations collaborate to evaluate and modify medicines as necessary.

9. Actual Information

Treatment choices are aided by real-world data, such as details on the efficacy of interventions in individuals infected with various strains.

10. The significance of immunization:

While Paxlovid and other antiviral medications are essential for treating COVID-19, immunization is still the most effective method for preventing infection and transmission, including from variations.

The general incidence of the virus can be lowered and the generation of new varieties can be constrained with widespread immunization.

In conclusion, the genetic makeup of particular SARS-CoV-2 variants determines how well Paxlovid works against those variations. For evaluating how well it performs against newly developing variations and for modifying treatment plans as necessary, ongoing study and surveillance are crucial. The creation and use of antiviral medications like Paxlovid should be viewed as a component of a larger COVID-19 defense strategy that also involves immunization, public health initiatives, and continual surveillance of the virus's growth.

PAXLOVID MANUFACTURING AND DEVELOPMENT

A number of processes in the development, testing, and manufacture go into the creation of Paxlovid, an antiviral drug used to treat COVID-19. Here is a thorough explanation of how Paxlovid is developed and produced:

Preclinical testing and drug discovery:

Drug discovery, which is the first step in the development process, involves the identification of candidate substances that may have antiviral activities against SARS-CoV-2.

Candidates that show promise are put through preclinical testing on animals and in labs to determine their safety and effectiveness.

2. Medical Research:

Clinical trials on humans are next for promising substances like nirmatrelvir and ritonavir, which are the active ingredients in Paxlovid. There are numerous phases to these trials:

Phase 1: Miniature studies to evaluate the dosage and safety in healthy individuals.

Phase 2: Larger studies with people who have the targeted ailment are conducted to further assess safety and efficacy.

Phase 3: Extensive studies to validate safety and effectiveness in a broad population. For COVID-19, Paxlovid underwent Phase 3 trials. 3. Regulatory Review:

Pharmaceutical firms submit their data to regulatory organizations like the U.S. Food and Drug Administration (FDA) for approval or Emergency Use Authorization (EUA) in the event of a pandemic after successful clinical trials.
Scaling Up Manufacturing:

Pharmaceutical businesses increase production to satisfy demand after receiving regulatory approval. Increasing production capacity is necessary for this.
To make Paxlovid on a bigger scale, businesses may employ their own manufacturing facilities or contract manufacturing organizations (CMOs).
5. Quality Assurance:

To guarantee the integrity, efficacy, and uniformity of every batch of Paxlovid, quality control procedures are rigorous. This entails thorough testing of the end product, intermediates, and raw components. Packaging and formulation:

The final dosage form of paxlovid is created; commonly, tablets. The drug's formulation guarantees its effectiveness, stability, and simplicity of administration.

After that, the finished item is put into the proper packaging for distribution.

7. Supply chain and distribution:

Paxlovid must be delivered to healthcare facilities, pharmacies, and authorized distribution sites via distributors and supply chain partners.

Distribution systems are set up to provide prompt availability to the drug.

8. Post-Market Monitoring

Pharmacovigilance programs continue to check Paxlovid for safety and efficacy in real-world situations even after it has been approved and made available.

9. Worldwide Cooperation:

Due to the pandemic's global reach, international cooperation is crucial. Governments, pharmaceutical firms, and regulatory bodies collaborate to guarantee Paxlovid distribution and access globally.

10. Modifications for Alternatives

Pharmaceutical companies and researchers may need to modify

antiviral medications like Paxlovid to maintain their efficacy against changing strains of SARS-CoV-2 as new variants appear.

Like any pharmaceutical product, Paxlovid's research and production are subject to stringent regulations to guarantee its safety and effectiveness. In order to give patients effective medicines and combat the COVID-19 pandemic, this method is defined by collaboration between researchers, regulatory authorities, pharmaceutical corporations, and healthcare professionals.

PAXLOVID PATIENT EXPERIENCES

Paxlovid was a relatively new drug for the treatment of COVID-19 at the time of my most recent knowledge update in September 2021, and there may not have been many patient experiences with it. However, based on the knowledge that was available at the time, I may offer some insights into what patients might anticipate when taking Paxlovid:

1. Early Intervention Is Vital:

When given early in COVID-19, ideally within the first few days of symptom manifestation, pax ovid is most helpful. Patients who think they may have COVID-19 should get tested

right away and consult a doctor to see if Paxlovid is the best course of action.
2. A decrease in symptoms

The symptoms of COVID-19 may lessen in patients who take Paxlovid. This may involve a decline in the virus' typical symptoms, such as fever, coughing, exhaustion, and others.
3. Shorter Illness Duration:

Paxlovid is designed to lessen the length of illness and stop the development of serious disease. When given Paxlovid, patients may heal more quickly than those who do not take antiviral medication.
4. Possible negative effects

Paxlovid, like all medicines, may cause negative effects. In clinical trials, the most frequent side effects were diarrhoea and nausea. Additionally, some individuals may develop skin rashes.

Patients should inform their healthcare practitioner of any adverse effects so that they can receive advice on how to manage them.

5. Treatment Compliance:

When taking Paxlovid, patients must adhere to their doctor's recommendations, including the suggested dosage and course of treatment. For the treatment to be as successful as possible, the entire course must be completed.

6. Follow-Up and Monitoring:

The effectiveness of the drug should be evaluated, and patients using Paxlovid should have their symptoms checked often by their doctor to make sure they are getting better.

To monitor progress, follow-up appointments or telemedicine sessions may be planned.

7. Possible Effects on Hospitalization

Early administration of paxlovid has been proven to lower the risk of COVID-19-related hospitalization. Particularly if they are at a higher risk for developing a serious illness, patients should be aware of this potential advantage.

8. Continued Safety Measures:

Patients should continue to adhere to public health recommendations, such as mask use, physical seclusion, and hand hygiene, even when taking Paxlovid, to stop the virus from spreading to others.

9. Support for Patients:

Patients with COVID-19 may feel stressed or anxious as a result of their condition. Healthcare professionals may provide patients with information and support to help them maintain their mental and emotional health during their sickness and recovery.

It's vital to remember that Paxlovid's accessibility and prescription requirements may differ by location and change over time. To get the most recent information about COVID-19 treatments, including Paxlovid, and to talk about their specific treatment plan, side effects, and other issues, patients should always speak with their healthcare professional. It's essential to consult the most recent data and research because patient experiences and knowledge of Paxlovid might have changed since my previous knowledge update.

INFLUENCE OF PAXLOVID ON VIRAL TRANSMISSION

Paxlovid's effect on viral transmission relates to how the drug may influence how SARS-CoV-2, the virus that causes COVID-19, spreads across populations and communities. The potential effect of Paxlovid on viral transmission is described in more depth below:

1. Lowering the viral load

Paxlovid is an antiviral drug that specifically attacks the SARS-CoV-2 virus. It functions by preventing the virus's capacity to multiply inside the cells of the body.
Paxlovid may be able to reduce the viral load in infected people by

inhibiting viral replication. A decreased viral load indicates that there are fewer virus particles in the mucus and saliva found in infected people's respiratory secretions.

2. The effect on infection transmission from infected people:

People who have a reduced viral load can be less infectious. When speaking, sneezing, or coughing, they may expel fewer virus particles, decreasing the likelihood that they will spread the illness to close contacts.

Early Intervention and Transmission:

When given early in COVID-19, ideally within the first few days of symptom manifestation, pax ovid is most helpful.

Rapid Paxlovid administration to infected patients can aid in lowering viral replication and transmission risk at an early stage of illness.

4. Benefit to public health:

Paxlovid can aid in the larger public health campaign to stop the spread of COVID-19 by lowering transmission potential.

Lower transmission rates lessen the strain on healthcare systems, safeguard vulnerable populations, and prevent the spread of the pandemic.

5. Coupling Techniques:

Paxlovid can be used as part of a complete plan to stop the spread of viruses by combining it with other public health measures like immunization, testing, contact tracing, and quarantine.

6. Impact on Alternatives:

If the many SARS-CoV-2 variants are sensitive to paxlovid, it may be able to lessen viral transmission because the drug's effect on viral replication is not variant-specific.

7. Impacts on the populace

The efficiency of the drug, the proportion of sick people who receive treatment, and adherence to treatment recommendations all play a role in how much Paxlovid affects viral transmission at the population level.

8. Limitations and Challenges:

It's vital to remember that Paxlovid is not a standalone remedy, even though it may be able to lower viral transmission. Other strategies, including immunization, mask use, physical separation, and hand hygiene, are also essential in decreasing transmission.

The effectiveness of Paxlovid in preventing the spread of infection is largely dependent on its accessibility and availability, as well as on the speed with which sick people can be located and treated.

9. Research and observation:

To evaluate Paxlovid's effect on viral transmission in various groups and contexts, further study and data collecting from actual situations are required.

In conclusion, Paxlovid's capacity to lessen viral propagation is a crucial component of its function in controlling the COVID-19 pandemic. Although the drug may assist lower viral load and lessen the likelihood of transmission, it should be taken into account as part of a larger plan that also involves vaccination, public health measures, and continuous study to comprehend its actual effects on transmission dynamics. Based on developing information and evidence about medications like Paxlovid, public health authorities and healthcare practitioners will continue to evaluate and adapt COVID-19 management options.

PAXLOVID'S EFFECTS ON THE HEALTHCARE SYSTEM AND THE ECONOMY

There are numerous effects on the economy and the healthcare system from the development and use of Paxlovid, an antiviral drug for the treatment of COVID-19. These consequences are explained in more depth below:

1. Effects on the economy:

Cost of Medicine (a)

Paxlovid's price may have a big impact on the economy. The cost of the medication, which can vary by area and healthcare system, may have an impact on access to therapy.

b. Lessened Financial Burden:

The financial cost of the COVID-19 pandemic may be lessened with the use of effective medications like Paxlovid. These therapies can cut healthcare expenditures and free up hospital resources by lowering hospital stays and serious cases.

Effect on Productivity: c

Paxlovid can aid people in recovering from COVID-19 more quickly. By lowering the number of sick days, this can boost labor productivity and promote financial stability.

Cost-Effectiveness Research:

Paxlovid's worth in terms of the advantages it offers in comparison to its price may be evaluated economically through studies like cost-effectiveness analyses.

2. Implications for the Healthcare System:

Reduced Hospitalization:

It has been demonstrated that paxlovid lowers the likelihood of hospitalization in people with COVID-19. This can ease the load that high hospitalization rates are putting on healthcare systems.

b. Resource Distribution

The distribution of resources across healthcare systems may be influenced by Paxlovid's accessibility. If hospitalizations decline, hospitals might need to devote fewer resources to COVID-19 patients.

b. Treatment Recommendations:

To include Paxlovid as a therapy option for COVID-19, healthcare systems and professional organizations may need to revise their treatment protocols. d. Healthcare Worker Protection:

Frontline workers' risk of infection can be decreased by using effective therapies like Paxlovid to shield them from prolonged virus exposure.
f. Outpatient Care and Telehealth:

The fact that Paxlovid is a medication that may be used for outpatient therapy may encourage the use of telehealth and outpatient care, easing the pressure on emergency rooms and inpatient institutions.
f. Distribution and pharmacies:

In order to guarantee that Paxlovid reaches patients in a timely and secure manner, healthcare organizations need effective distribution and pharmacy management.

3. Considerations for Equity:

Access Inequalities:

To prevent escalating healthcare inequities, it is critical to guarantee equitable access to Paxlovid. Reaching marginalized and vulnerable people requires effort.

Financial Obstacles:

Access to Paxlovid may be hampered by financial obstacles such high prescription costs or a lack of insurance coverage. There should be plans in place to remove these obstacles.

Pharmacy monitoring:

Pharmacovigilance systems are necessary in healthcare systems to keep an eye on Paxlovid's efficacy and safety in practical situations. This includes documenting and keeping track of negative incidents.

5. Public Health Communications

To inform the general public and healthcare professionals about the availability and recommended use of Paxlovid, clear and accurate public health messaging is crucial.

6. Pandemic Preparedness in the Future:

The launch of Paxlovid emphasizes the significance of including antiviral medications in pandemic preparedness strategies. Future techniques for storing and distributing these drugs may need to be developed by healthcare systems.

In conclusion, Paxlovid has important consequences for the economy and healthcare system. While it would lessen the load on healthcare institutions and the financial burden of the COVID-19 epidemic, it also raises issues with access, distribution, and pricing. Addressing these consequences, ensuring equitable access, and tracking its effects on patient outcomes and healthcare system dynamics are all necessary for effective management of the introduction of Paxlovid.

PAXLOVID AND CONCERNING VARIANTS

In the ongoing fight against the pandemic, paxlovid's interaction with Variants of Concern (VOCs) of SARS-CoV-2, the virus that produces COVID-19, is crucial to take into account. The relationship between Paxlovid and VOCs is explained in more detail below:

1. VOCs: Variants of Concern

VOCs are special SARS-CoV-2 virus strains that have undergone changes to important parts of their genetic makeup, particularly the spike protein. These alterations may affect a virus's capacity to spread, dodge immune responses, and perhaps even be vulnerable to drugs and vaccinations.

2. The effect of variations on therapies:

Theoretically, the genetic alterations in VOCs could affect how well medications like Paxlovid, which target particular steps in the viral replication process, work.

Since many antiviral medications and neutralizing antibodies target the spike protein mutations, they are particularly important.

3. Research in the Lab:

To determine how effectively medications like Paxlovid combat particular VOCs, researchers conduct laboratory experiments.

These investigations examine the efficiency of the medication against viral samples that have the mutations seen in VOCs.

4. Possible Modifications:

Pharmaceutical companies may need to modify the formulation or dosage of medications like Paxlovid if laboratory tests point to decreased potency against specific VOCs.

Drug producers and regulatory organizations keep an eye on how well therapies work against new variations.

5. Concurrent Therapies:

To improve the efficacy of treatment against various variations, healthcare providers may occasionally consider combination therapies that involve multiple medications with distinct mechanisms of action.

Real-World Information:

Treatment choices are influenced by real-world data, such as information on the efficacy of interventions in patients exposed to various VOCs.

7. Sequencing and surveillance

Understanding how the virus is changing and whether it affects treatment and vaccine responses requires ongoing surveillance and genetic sequencing of SARS-CoV-2 variants.

Monitoring aids in the detection of VOCs and variations with particular dangerous alterations.

8. Quick Reaction

Rapid treatment adaptation, such what is possible with Paxlovid, to deal with novel VOCs, is a crucial component of pandemic response.

Pharmaceutical firms and regulatory organizations collaborate to evaluate and modify medicines as necessary.

9. The significance of immunization:

While Paxlovid and other antiviral medications are essential for treating COVID-19, immunization is still one of the most effective ways to stop infection and transmission, including those caused by VOCs.

The general incidence of the virus can be lowered and the generation of new varieties can be constrained with widespread immunization.

Influence on Public Health: 10.

The potential negative effects of VOCs on treatment outcomes highlight the significance of taking preventative measures including immunization, mask use, and physical separation to stop the virus from spreading.

In short, the genetic make-up of those variants determines how well Paxlovid works against particular VOCs. In order to evaluate how well a treatment strategy performs against newly emerging variations and to adjust it as necessary, ongoing research, surveillance, and adaptation efforts are crucial. The creation and use of antiviral medications like Paxlovid should be viewed as a component of a larger COVID-19 prevention strategy that also involves immunization, public health initiatives, and continual surveillance of the virus's evolution and its effects on available treatments.

PAXLOVID AND IMMUNIZATION PLANS

A key component of thorough pandemic management is the incorporation of antiviral drugs like Paxlovid with immunization programs. Here is where Paxlovid fits into immunization plans:

Complementary Strategy:

Antiviral drugs like Paxlovid offer an extra line of defense against COVID-19, particularly for people who cannot receive the vaccination owing to a medical condition or who are not yet eligible, such as young children. They are also a form of treatment for those who get the virus despite receiving the vaccine.
**2. Care for Innovative Cases:

Infections can emerge despite the effectiveness of immunizations. When someone gets immunized but still contracts COVID-19, they may be treated with paxlovid, especially if they are at a high risk of developing a serious illness.

Relieving Pressure on Healthcare Systems:

Paxlovid and comparable antivirals lessen the strain on healthcare systems by lowering the severity of disease, allowing them to concentrate more on vaccination campaigns and other urgent healthcare requirements.

**4. Increasing Vaccination Confidence:

Public confidence in COVID-19 vaccines may increase knowing that viable therapies are available. If people are aware that there are effective therapies available in case they still get the virus, they may be more willing to be vaccinated.

5. Offering a Safety Net

Antiviral drugs serve as a safety net, assuring that, even if someone acquires COVID-19 after vaccination, there will be treatments that can dramatically lower the risk of serious illness and hospitalization.

Possibility of Post-Exposure Prophylaxis (**6):

Antiviral drugs may be used as post-exposure prophylaxis, especially for those who have had intimate contact with someone who has been diagnosed with COVID-19. By doing this, the infection might not turn into a serious sickness.

**7. Variant Adaptation:

Some SARS-CoV-2 variations may partially circumvent vaccine-induced immunity as new SARS-CoV-2 variants develop. If the antiviral drug is still effective against the variations, it may be possible to treat instances involving variants using it.

Global Immunization Equity: **8.

Antiviral medicines like Paxlovid can be a crucial alternative for controlling COVID-19 cases and lessening the effect of the virus in these communities in areas where vaccination rates are low due to restricted access or vaccine reluctance.

**9. Studying Combined Methods:

In order to understand how these methods can cooperate to lessen the spread of COVID-19 and severe illness, ongoing research examines the effectiveness of combining vaccinations and antiviral drugs.

In order to maximize the overall effect on containing the pandemic, public health institutions continuously assess the effectiveness of vaccines and antiviral treatments and alter strategies as necessary based on actual facts.

In conclusion, combining antiviral drugs like Paxlovid with vaccination plans gives a complex strategy for controlling the COVID-19 pandemic. Healthcare systems can better protect populations, ease the pressure on hospitals, and ultimately save lives by combining immunization campaigns with efficient treatments. To best utilize vaccines and antiviral drugs in the fight against COVID-19, ongoing research and collaboration between medical professionals, researchers, and politicians are crucial.

PATIENT AWARENESS AND EDUCATION

In order to give patients the knowledge and understanding they need to actively participate in their own treatment, patient education and awareness are essential elements of healthcare delivery. Here is a thorough examination of patient awareness and education:

Recognizing Medical Conditions:

Understanding certain medical diseases, their causes, symptoms, and potential remedies is the first step in patient education. Patients must be given concise, jargon-free explanations in order to fully understand the nature of their sickness.

**2. Available Therapies:

The numerous therapy options that are available to patients must be made clear to them. This covers not just conventional medical interventions like drugs and operations but also potentially helpful alternative therapies or way of life adjustments.

**3. Instruction in Medication:

Patients must fully comprehend the medications that have been recommended to them. This includes being aware of the medication's intended use, the proper dosage, any possible adverse effects, and the best way to take the medication (with food, without food, at particular times, etc.).

**4. Making Knowledgeable Decisions:

Patients who are well-informed can take an active role in selecting their treatments. In order to enable patients to make well-informed decisions, healthcare practitioners should provide adequate information regarding various treatment options, possible results, and dangers.

Preventive measures and a healthy lifestyle:

Patients can considerably improve their general well-being and lower their chance of getting certain disorders by learning about preventative measures and the value of leading a healthy lifestyle (diet, exercise, stress management).

**Diagnostic Procedures and Tests:

Any diagnostic treatments or tests that the patient's healthcare professional suggests should be disclosed to the patient. This covers the need for the test, how it's carried out, and what the outcomes might show.

**7. Taking Care of Chronic Illnesses:

Effective self-care for patients with chronic illnesses depends on their knowledge of their illness, long-term treatment techniques, and potential complications.

**8. Care Following Treatment:

Patients require detailed information on how to care for themselves after procedures or treatments. This could involve managing medications, treating wounds, and spotting complications.

**10. Physical and Mental Health:

Mental health should be covered in patient education, along with symptoms of mental health illnesses, coping mechanisms, and the significance of getting treatment when you need it.

10. Utilizing Technology: - Patient education can be improved by using wearable tech, apps, and websites for healthcare. These resources can include self-management tools, medication reminders, and individualized health information.

Healthcare professionals should speak in a way that patients can comprehend, taking into account their varied origins and literacy levels. It should be easy for patients to ask questions regarding their health.

Support Systems: - Providing patients with information about support groups, counseling services, and community resources helps foster a sense of community and emotional support, especially for those managing chronic conditions.

Preventing False Information: - Patients frequently look online for health information in the internet age. It's critical to point patients toward trustworthy resources and caution against false information that could cause needless concern or erroneous self-diagnosis.

**14. Culturally Competent Education: - To guarantee awareness and respect for individual variations, patient education materials and discussions should be culturally competent, taking into account various beliefs, languages, and customs.

Patient education is not a one-time event; rather, it involves ongoing communication between patients and healthcare professionals. Patients can address worries and anxieties right away thanks to frequent follow-ups and clear lines of contact.

The foundational pillars of patient-centered care are patient education and awareness, to sum up. Healthcare professionals can empower their patients to take an active role in their health and enhance outcomes as well as general well-being by giving them accurate, understandable, and culturally sensitive information.

MANUFACTURING AND SUPPLY CHAIN ISSUES WITH PAXLOVID

An elaborate and complicated process goes into producing and supplying a breakthrough pharmaceutical product like Paxlovid. Paxlovid's manufacturing and supply chain may face the following difficulties:

**1. Scale-Up Obstacles

It can be difficult to scale up manufacturing to meet the demand for Paxlovid on a global scale. The necessity for manufacturing facility expansion by pharmaceutical companies necessitates a large financial, time, and resource commitment.

**2. Sourcing of Raw Materials:

It's crucial to guarantee a consistent supply of superior raw materials. The production process can be stopped by any supply chain disturbances, such as shortages or poor-quality raw materials.

**3. Manufacturing of Active Pharmaceutical Ingredients (API):

Paxlovid's API, or active pharmaceutical ingredient, is produced using intricate procedures. For the medicine to be effective and safe, the consistency, quality, and purity of the API must be guaranteed.

Quality Assurance and Control:

To adhere to regulatory requirements, high quality control and assurance standards must be maintained. For patient safety, it is essential that each batch of Paxlovid meets quality requirements.

**5. Adherence to Regulations:

It might take a long time and be difficult to gain the appropriate permissions and to comply with regulatory standards in many nations. Good Manufacturing Practices (GMP) compliance is necessary and necessitates strict documentation and adherence to rules.

**Requirements for the Cold Chain

Paxlovid and other medicinal goods may need particular temperature management throughout the supply chain. It is essential to maintain the cold chain's integrity, particularly during shipment and storage.

Packaging and labeling **7.

Regulations must be followed, and packaging and labeling must be harmonized for different markets. It is crucial to make sure that the packaging safeguards the product and gives precise dose instructions.

**8. Difficulties in Global Distribution

Global Paxlovid distribution requires a well-organized logistics network. Customs laws, transportation restrictions, and the requirement for effective distribution facilities are issues.

**9. Variability in Demand:

There may be regional and temporal variations in the demand for Paxlovid. To prevent shortages or overstocking, pharmaceutical businesses must prepare for these swings and adapt their strategies.

**10. Intellectual Property and Collaboration: - Paxlovid's accessibility and cost may be impacted by intellectual property difficulties, such as patent disputes and partnerships with generic producers in underdeveloped nations.

Manufacturing, transportation, and distribution can all be impacted by supply chain disruptions, such as those caused by natural catastrophes, political unrest, or public health events (like the COVID-19 pandemic).

**12. Equitable Distribution: - It is difficult to guarantee that Paxlovid is accessible to everyone, including in low-income nations. In areas with little resources, efforts must be made to ensure availability and prevent inequities.

Pharmacovigilance is the process of evaluating a drug's safety and effectiveness after it has been put on the market. To keep track of adverse events, a strong pharmacovigilance system must be established.

Taking into account New Variants: - There may be a need for modifications to the production procedure or formulations as new COVID-19 viral variations appear to ensure Paxlovid's efficacy against these versions.

Pharmaceutical firms, regulatory bodies, logistical partners, and international organizations must work together to address these issues. To guarantee a steady and dependable supply of Paxlovid to patients globally, proactive planning, investment in production capacities, adherence to quality standards, and effective supply chain management are essential.

THE FUNCTION OF PAXLOVID IN PANDEMIC PREPAREDNESS

Paxlovid is a key component of pandemic preparedness plans as an antiviral drug for COVID-19. Here is how Paxlovid helps with pandemic readiness:

Early symptom management and treatment:

When given early in the course of the illness to individuals with mild to moderate COVID-19 symptoms, paxlovid has been demonstrated to be particularly beneficial at lowering the risk of hospitalization and mortality. By stopping the spread of cases, this can ease the burden on healthcare systems during a pandemic.

Reducing Hospitalizations and Severity:

Paxlovid can decrease the number of hospitalizations and admissions to intensive care by lessening the severity of disease. This is critical during a pandemic since hospitals frequently deal with a large patient load.

3. Vulnerable Populations Protection:

The risk of developing a serious illness from COVID-19 is higher in vulnerable populations, such as the elderly and people with existing medical issues. Paxlovid offers an extra layer of defense for these people, possibly lowering mortality rates in high-risk groups.

**4. Worldwide Distribution and Stockpiling:

Countries can store Paxlovid and other antiviral drugs as part of their pandemic preparedness efforts. In the case of an outbreak, these stores serve as a tactical reserve that may be quickly deployed, assuring prompt access to care.

**5. Adaptable Reaction to Variants:

The development of novel viral strains frequently occurs during pandemics. Antiviral drugs like Paxlovid, which may be modified or tested to assure effectiveness against various variations, can offer a flexible response. Being adaptable is essential for avoiding the infection.

**6. Avoiding Transmission in Situations at High Risk:

Paxlovid can be used proactively to manage outbreaks and lower transmission in high-risk environments where preventing the spread of the virus can be difficult, such as long-term care institutions, prisons, or highly populated places.

Combination with a vaccine: **7

Paxlovid can offer prompt treatment for breakthrough infections in conjunction with vaccination campaigns, ensuring that those who have received the vaccine have access to efficient treatments should they still develop the virus.

**8. Lessening the Financial Impact:

Paxlovid can help lessen the financial toll of a pandemic by minimizing serious sickness and hospitalisation.

The economy will indirectly benefit from fewer hospitalizations since there will be less of a burden on healthcare resources and cheaper healthcare expenses.

**9. Education and Public Health Messaging:

Paxlovid's accessibility is included in public health messaging as well. It can boost public confidence and promote adherence to advised preventative measures and immunization campaigns to know that an effective cure is available.

**10. Incentives for Research and Development: Antiviral drugs like Paxlovid exist, which encourages more study and advancement in the sector. Researchers and pharmaceutical companies are urged to keep working to provide even more potent medicines for upcoming pandemics.

In conclusion, Paxlovid has a variety of functions in pandemic readiness. In particular for vulnerable populations, it provides a crucial tool for preventing serious disease and hospitalisation. It improves healthcare systems' ability to manage cases, lowers mortality rates, and helps create a more robust and efficient response to upcoming pandemics when integrated into complete pandemic response plans.

RESEARCH ON PAXLOVID IN THE FUTURE

Future directions for Paxlovid research would probably focus on a few important areas in order to maximize its effectiveness, safety, and accessibility as of my most recent update in September 2021. Here are some probable directions for Paxlovid's future research:

Long-term safety and effectiveness:

ongoing evaluation of the safety and effectiveness of Paxlovid over the long term in patients who have had it for extended periods. In order to comprehend any potential delayed side effects and guarantee the drug's long-term safety profile, long-term trials are essential.

**2. Concurrent Therapies:

investigation on the efficacy of combining Paxlovid with additional antiviral treatments or immune-modulating therapies. Combination therapy may improve overall efficacy, particularly in people with severe COVID-19 or those whose immune systems have been damaged.

**3. Use and safety in children:

Clinical studies examining the Paxlovid safety and effectiveness in pediatric patients. It is crucial to comprehend how Paxlovid interacts with developing bodies before using it on youngsters, who are similarly prone to severe COVID-19 cases.

**4. Improving Administration and Dosage:

Paxlovid dosage, method of administration, and treatment length research. For both inpatient and outpatient settings, determining the most practical and efficient dose schedule is crucial.
**5. Different Concerns:

Studying Paxlovid's efficacy against newly-emerging SARS-CoV-2 variants is crucial since the virus is prone to mutation, therefore continual study is necessary to make sure Paxlovid is still effective against new strains.
Post-Exposure Prophylaxis (**6)

examining Paxlovid's potential as a preventive post-exposure therapy. Giving Paxlovid to those who have had frequent contact with confirmed COVID-19 patients may stop the infection from developing into a serious illness.

**7. Accessibility and affordability globally

Paxlovid accessibility and cost-effectiveness research, particularly in low-income nations. To provide equitable access, this may entail working with governments, NGOs, and international organizations.

**8. Monitoring Resistance:

Keeping an eye on and investigating probable Paxlovid resistance cases. Future treatment plans can be influenced by an understanding of how resistance develops, and more potent antiviral medications can be created.

**9. Studies on Real-World Effectiveness:

To evaluate Paxlovid's effectiveness in various healthcare settings, real-world effectiveness studies are being conducted. Real-world statistics can offer insightful information regarding its practical use, adherence rates, and general efficacy.

Special Populations: **10. research that focuses on particular groups, like expectant mothers, people with weakened immune systems, and the elderly. In order to create individualized treatment regimens, it is essential to comprehend how Paxlovid interacts with particular medical disorders.

Comparative efficacy studies comparing Paxlovid to other antiviral drugs and therapies are referenced in item 11. These studies can aid medical professionals in selecting the most appropriate therapies for various patient populations.

**12. Mechanistic investigations: - Extensive mechanistic investigations to comprehend the cellular and molecular mechanisms underlying Paxlovid's action. The creation of more specialized antiviral treatments may be influenced by our understanding of its mechanics.

Research is being done to find a way to incorporate Paxlovid into worldwide pandemic preparedness strategies. This could entail developing frameworks for quick deployment, stockpiling plans, and global partnerships for a coordinated reaction.

It's important to remember that there may have been advances and ongoing study since my previous update. I suggest referring to current scientific articles, clinical trial databases, and updates from credible health organizations for the most up-to-date details on Paxlovid research.

Made in the USA
Las Vegas, NV
14 July 2024

92321385R00066